Your Guide to

Total Hip Replacement

Fairview Health Services

Minneapolis, Minnesota

Published by Fairview Press, 2450 Riverside Avenue, Minneapolis, Minnesota 55454. Fairview Press is a division of Fairview Health Services, a community-focused health system affiliated with the University of Minnesota and providing a complete range of services, from the prevention of illness and injury to care for the most complex medical conditions.

Library of Congress Cataloging-in-Publication Data
Your guide to total hip replacement / Fairview Health Services.
    p. cm.
  Includes bibliographical references (p.   )
  ISBN-13: 978-1-57749-164-4 (pbk. : alk. paper)
  ISBN-10: 1-57749-164-5 (pbk. : alk. paper)
  1. Total hip replacement--Popular works. I. Fairview Health Services.
  RD549.Y69 2007
  617.5'80592--dc22

                       2006021472

First Printing: January 2007
Printed in the United States of America
11 10 09 08 07   6 5 4 3 2 1

Illustrations by Laurie Ingram
Edited by Lee Engfer

Medical Disclaimer
This publication is designed to provide accurate and authoritative information in regard to the subject matter covered. It is sold with the understanding that the publisher is not engaged in the provision or practice of medical, nursing, or professional health care advice or services in any jurisdiction. If medical advice or other professional assistance is required, the services of a qualified and competent professional should be sought. Fairview Press is not responsible or liable, directly or indirectly, for any form of damages whatsoever resulting from the use (or misuse) of information contained in or implied by these documents.

Customized editions of this publication (imprinted with your institution's name, contact information, etc.) are also available. Contact Fairview Press at 612-672-4774 for pricing.

Contents

Introduction

Total hip replacement is surgery to replace a painful hip joint. The surgery can help you get back to doing the things you want to do.

As you get ready for surgery you may have a lot of questions. Many people find it helpful to learn as much as they can about total hip replacement. This book lets you know what to expect before, during and after surgery.

Fairview Health Services developed this book as a learning tool. Our goal is to give you basic facts about total hip replacement and help you plan for your surgery, hospital stay and recovery. This book also offers tips for living with your new hip. It will help you understand the goals you'll work toward and the guidelines for hip safety.

Please take some time to read the whole book before your surgery. You don't have to read it all at once—go at your own pace. If you have questions, ask your doctor or nurse.

Your health care team

Your health care team will work together during your surgery, hospital stay and recovery. You and your family are the most important members of your health care team. You will help your recovery by taking an active role in your care.

Along with your doctor and surgeon, members of your health care team include:

- **Nurses.** A team of nurses and support staff will help with your care plan before and after surgery. They talk with other care providers to make sure all parts of your care work together. They help with your daily activities (including exercises and walking), treatments, personal care, pain relief and planning for when you leave the hospital.

- **Physical therapists.** These team members are trained to help you move safely with your new hip. They will work with you to strengthen your muscles before and after surgery. Physical therapists will develop an exercise program for you and show you how to do the movements. They will also show you how to use a walker or crutches.

- **Occupational therapists.** These therapists will teach you how to dress, manage personal care and do household tasks safely with your new hip. They will show you how to use equipment you may need to perform these tasks, such as a raised toilet seat.

- **Social workers and care coordinators.** These team members help you and your family plan for when you leave the hospital. They can tell you about helpful resources and talk with you about your insurance, or health plan.

Please tell you care team if you need a language interpreter or are deaf or hard of hearing. You have the right to a trained medical interpreter who will help you talk with doctors and nurses.

You might also want to ask if spiritual support is available at your hospital. Most hospitals have chaplains who support a range of faith traditions. Or you may contact your own faith community for support.

Don't forget: You are the most important member of your health care team.

Chapter 1

What Is Hip Replacement?

Your hips provide a stable base of support for your body. They are strong enough to carry your body's full weight. They allow you to walk, climb stairs, bend and twist.

A painful hip makes it harder to enjoy an active life. A hip that is damaged or worn down can't take the daily demands it once did.

Total hip replacement is surgery to remove the parts of the hip that are damaged and replace them with new parts. This can ease your pain and get you moving again. Hip replacement is one of the most common and successful surgeries.

Understanding your hip

> The hip is a ball and socket joint. The ball is the large, round upper end of the thighbone (femur). This fits into a cuplike socket (acetabulum) on the outer side of your pelvis, or hipbone (ilium).

> The bones of the hip joint are covered with a layer of cartilage, a smooth, tough tissue that keeps the bones from rubbing together. (You've probably seen cartilage on the end of a chicken drumstick.) Muscles and ligaments (tough bands of tissue) surround the joint and hold the ball in place inside the socket.

A healthy hip

In a healthy hip, the ball and socket fit closely together. The cartilage is smooth. This cushions your hip joint and allows the ball to glide easily inside the socket. The hip joint moves smoothly and the muscles around it support your weight.

A normal, healthy hip

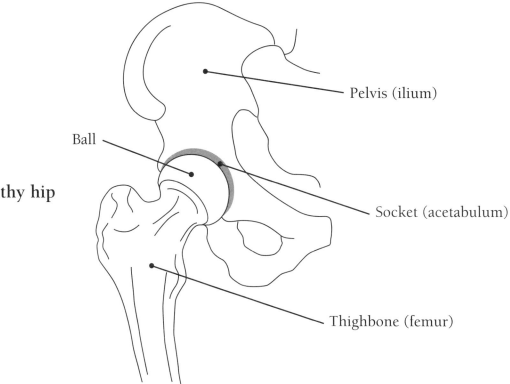

Pelvis (ilium)

Ball

Socket (acetabulum)

Thighbone (femur)

A painful hip

If your hip is hurt or worn down, the joint does not move smoothly. Movement becomes painful. You may have trouble putting weight on that leg. You might limp, and it may be hard to walk up or down stairs or stand up from a chair. A painful hip can keep you from doing the things you enjoy.

The most common reason for hip replacement is a disease called osteoarthritis (AHS-tee-oh-arth-RY-tuss). The cartilage wears away from the bones, causing the joint to lose its cushion. The surface of the bones becomes rough. As the hip moves, the ball of the hip joint grinds in the socket, causing pain and stiffness.

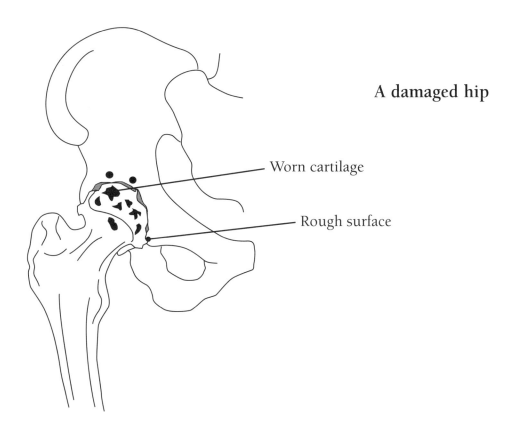

A damaged hip

— Worn cartilage

— Rough surface

As the pain gets worse, you may try to stop using your hip joint. This causes the muscles around the joint to weaken. People with arthritis in the hip have trouble walking, climbing stairs and doing simple things like tying shoes or clipping toenails.

Sometimes osteoarthritis occurs because of:

- A broken hip

- Childhood hip problems

- Past injuries that create extra wear and tear on the joint

- Rheumatoid (ROOM-uh-toyd) arthritis, a disease that causes stiffness, swelling and pain in the hip joints

- Loss of blood supply to the ball of the hip joint (called avascular necrosis). The bone in part of the ball dies and collapses. The ball becomes flat instead of round, and the hip joint does not move smoothly. This disease is often related to the use of steroids or alcohol, or to certain blood problems.

Getting a new hip

In total hip replacement surgery, doctors remove the ball and socket bones of the hip and thigh, along with damaged cartilage. They replace the joint with new parts made of metal, strong plastic or other material.

Surgery usually lasts two to three hours. A 6- to 8-inch cut (incision) is made to gain access to the hip joint. After removing the diseased bone, doctors prepare the remaining bone for the new joint. They may wedge the pieces tightly into place or fix them to the bone with a special cement. Your doctor will decide which method is best for you.

Some surgeons are doing hip replacements with one or two smaller incisions—sometimes referred to as "minimally invasive surgery." Recovery from these surgeries is somewhat different. The short-term benefits seem promising; the long-term risks and benefits are still being studied.

Minimally invasive surgery is a developing and evolving field. If you will be having this kind of surgery, please ask your surgeon which parts of this book apply to you.

The artificial hip

The artificial joint is called a prosthesis (PRAHSS-thee-sis). The ball is usually made of stainless steel or another long-lasting metal. The cup-shaped socket is usually made of metal and a very sturdy plastic.

These parts fit together to create a new hip with smooth surfaces. This makes for a natural, comfortable gliding motion.

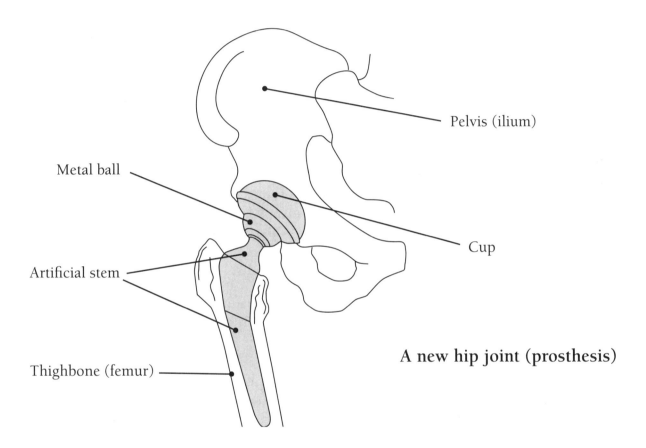

Pelvis (ilium)

Metal ball

Cup

Artificial stem

A new hip joint (prosthesis)

Thighbone (femur)

What to expect from surgery

The goal of hip replacement surgery is to reduce pain and stiffness. For most people, the surgery does just that.

Total hip replacement is one of the most successful joint operations. Long-term studies have shown pain relief in 90 to 95 percent of people who have this surgery.

After the pain from the surgery goes away, you will likely notice that your arthritis pain is gone, too. Most people have no ongoing pain, or they have a small amount that they control with over-the-counter medicine. People often feel less stiffness as well.

After healing, you'll be able to get back to many of the things you normally do, such as walking, biking, golfing, dancing and hiking. If you had low-back pain from the arthritis in your hip, you may find some relief from this as well.

In time, the joint may loosen and you may need another hip replacement. This can take as long as 20 years, though younger people may wear out their hips faster. Long-term results have improved as new techniques and parts have come into use.

The risks of surgery

Like any major surgery, hip replacement brings certain risks. Major problems, while uncommon, can be treated.

When a new hip fails, it is often due to infection or to loosening slowly over time (where the metal or cement meets the bone). Other common risks are:

- Different leg lengths

- Ball popping out of the socket (dislocation)

- Blood clots in the leg or lung

- Problems urinating (passing water when using the toilet)

- Nerve damage

Some of these problems happen soon after surgery. Others may not show up until years later.

Most problems can be prevented. Your health care team will show you how to move safely with your new hip and reduce the risk of problems. (See "Preventing complications," page 44.)

Questions to Ask Your Doctor

Before surgery, you will feel more prepared if you talk with your health care team and review this book. Be sure to ask:

- What are the short-term and long-term risks of this surgery?

- What can I do to get ready for surgery?

- Can I take my medicines before surgery?

- How long will it take for me to recover?

- When can I start driving again?

- When can I go back to work?

- What kind of help do you think I'll need in the first couples weeks after surgery?

Write down any other questions you have so you don't forget to ask them.

Chapter 2

Planning Ahead for Your Recovery

After hip surgery, it may be several months before you can do all the things you are used to doing. You can make this time easier by planning ahead.

The time to make plans for leaving the hospital is *before* you go in for surgery. The more ready you are, the more smoothly things will go at the hospital and at home. This chapter offers several tips to make recovery easier.

Make a recovery plan

Most people stay in the hospital for three nights after surgery. Your health care team will help you form a plan for leaving the hospital (called a discharge plan). This plan is based on your needs, your progress in using your new hip and your insurance coverage.

During your hospital stay, you will work toward a number of goals, such as getting in and out of bed safely and walking with your walker, crutches or cane. Your health care team will let you know if you can go straight home from the hospital or if you will need extra help.

Home

You can go home after leaving the hospital if you can:

- Get in and out of bed and a chair by yourself or with a little help from a caregiver.

- Walk with your walker, crutches or cane.

- Walk the distance from your bedroom to your bathroom and kitchen.

- Safely get on and off the toilet by yourself or with a little help.

- Go up and down stairs safely.

At home you will need help from family and friends for several weeks. You may need help with dressing, personal care and household tasks.

Your energy level will be lower than usual. Over time, you will need less help. If you are going right home after surgery, ask a family member, friend or neighbor to stay close by for the first week. If you live alone or are alone during the day, plan for someone to stay with you for at least the first few days to a week. Decide who will take you home from the hospital and drive you to doctor visits.

Home with home health services

If you can go home but will need more help, you may qualify for home health services. In this case, nurses, home health aides or physical or occupational therapists will visit you at home. They can help you with walking, strengthening exercises, daily activities and safety issues. They will also keep track of your overall health.

Your care team will let you know if you need these services. Talk with a social worker or care coordinator at the hospital to see if your insurance plan covers home health visits.

Tip

Arrange for a friend or family member to stay with you for the first week after surgery.

If you already use home health services, bring the agency's name and phone number to the hospital. Your social worker or care coordinator can help increase the amount of care you will receive at home. If you have not used home health services in the past, ask your care coordinator to help you find a home health agency.

Skilled nursing facility

Some people need more services than they can get at home. If this is true for you, you may need to spend a week or longer in a skilled nursing facility. (This is sometimes called an extended care facility, transitional care unit or "step-down" care facility.) Caregivers there will attend to your medical needs until you can safely return home. You will also get physical therapy every day. Therapy will help you build your strength and self-care skills. The care team will work with you and your family so you can go home as quickly as possible.

Your social worker or care coordinator can help you find a place that offers the short-term care you need. Try to find three facilities where you would feel comfortable. Call your insurance company to find out if these places are covered under your plan.

Understand your health insurance coverage

Health care benefits differ from one plan to another, and benefits often change. Before you have surgery, be sure you know what your insurance plan covers. Call your health plan or look at your policy book. Find out exactly what is and is not covered after surgery. Ask about home health care, a skilled nursing facility and medical equipment.

Tip

Know what your insurance plan will pay for. Ask about home health care, a skilled nursing facility and medical equipment.

Make a living will

A health care directive (also called an advance directive or living will) lets you decide what medical care you would want if you became unable to communicate. It tells your family about your wishes for treatment, such as whether you would want to be on a life-support machine.

A health care directive is useful for all adults, even those who are not facing major surgery. It is a written, legal document. Your family and medical team will turn to the directive if you become unable to make your own health care decisions.

Bring a copy of your health care directive to the hospital. It will be part of your files. If you don't have a health care directive, you may wish to ask for the forms you need to make a living will.

Plan for less activity

Your schedule will need to change after surgery, as you will not be able to do as much. Your movements and energy level will be limited. Let people know you will be "out of action" for a while. If you work, arrange for time off for the surgery and recovery. Talk to your health care team about how long you will need to be away from work.

Prepare your home

Tip

Set up a recovery station—the place where you will spend the most time after surgery. Keep the things you will use most within easy reach.

Another important step is to make your home safe and easy for you to get around. After surgery, you won't be able to bend over or reach up high. You will need to avoid twisting while sitting down, since this may cause your hip to dislocate.

These limits can make it hard to do things you take for granted, like bending down to grab a bar of soap that has fallen on the floor. Cooking and cleaning bring new challenges. Even something as simple as watching TV requires thought about where you keep the remote and whether you have to bend down to use a VCR or DVD player.

Before surgery, make your home as accessible as possible. Follow the tips on page 14 ("Getting your home ready for your return"). Set up a "recovery station" where you will spend most of your time. You should be able to reach it without twisting. In this handy spot, keep the things you use most—the TV remote control, phone, medicine, books, magazines, reading glasses, tissues, waste basket, a pitcher of water and a glass for drinking.

Stock up on basic groceries and meals that are quick and easy to make. It's a good idea to prepare some meals in advance and freeze them. Frozen casseroles and soups can be reheated and served easily.

Talk to a physical or occupational therapist about equipment you may need to install in your home. You may rent or buy items that make it easier for you to use the bathtub, toilet and other areas. For a list of items that can help, see chapter 5.

If You Live Alone

Before you go to the hospital, ask your health care team how to set up your home to make your tasks easier. You will need someone to stay with you for the first few days to a week. After that, think about the tasks you will need help with. Ask family and friends for help with the things you can't do on your own.

Here are some things to think about if you live alone.

- Find someone to help care for your pet while you're in the hospital.

- Ask a neighbor to do your outdoor work, such as lawn mowing or shoveling, while you are healing.

- Make plans to have someone drive you to the grocery store, religious services, family events and doctor and therapy visits. Keep a list of people who are willing to take turns helping out.

- If you don't have many people to help you, talk with your social worker or care coordinator. He or she can put you in touch with resources in your area.

Getting Your Home Ready for Your Return

General

- Leave your home clean and tidy so you won't have to clean it when you return.

- Keep a phone near your bed and main living area. Post emergency numbers on or near the phones. When you are home alone, carry a cordless or mobile phone.

- Make sure you have a chair with a firm seat and arms. You will not be able to sit in a recliner, soft chair, rocking chair or sofa for at least six weeks after surgery. A good chair is high and firm enough to allow your feet to be flat on the floor and your knees to be lower than your hips.

- Keep items that you use often at arm level so you don't have to reach up or bend down.

- Remove throw rugs. Tape down the edges of large area rugs.

- Remove clutter from hallways and other pathways. Keep walkways free of furniture, electrical cords and phone cords.

- If you have stairs in your home, make sure there is a handrail. Check railings to make sure they are not wobbly. If you are adding a new handrail, it should extend a few inches past the end of the staircase.

- Be sure you have enough light indoors, outdoors and in stairways. Put night-lights in dark hallways.

- Ask your mail and newspaper carriers to deliver to your door. If you can, have packages and newspapers placed on a bench, rather than the floor.

Getting Your Home Ready for Your Return

Bedroom

- Do not use a waterbed. Use a regular bed with a box spring and mattress. If your bed is upstairs, you might want to move it to the main floor for the weeks of recovery.

- Leave extra space around your bed. This gives you room to get in and out while using crutches, a walker or a cane.

- Keep a flashlight next to your bed. Or, use night-lights for nighttime trips to the bathroom.

Bathroom

- Install a raised toilet seat. (See page 58.)

- Use a rubber mat or nonskid tape strips in the bathtub or shower stall. This helps prevent falls.

- If your bathroom is not on the main floor where you're sleeping, look into getting a commode, or portable toilet. (See page 58.)

- Put grab bars in the bathtub or shower. You may also need grab bars by the toilet.

- Install a hand-held showerhead to make bathing easier. (See page 59.)

- Liquid soap may be easier to use than bar soap, which can slip away.

Kitchen

- Use a cart to move heavy or hot items.

- Place utensils where you can reach them without bending or stretching.

- It may be hard to use the dishwasher. Instead, use a dish drainer in the sink or on the counter.

- Plan to use the microwave for cooking. If you want to use the stove, leave saucepans on the stove or at stovetop height.

Recovery plan timeline

It will take several weeks to plan your recovery and get ready for surgery. While everyone's needs are different, these are the basic steps you will need to take.

6 weeks before surgery

Tip

Schedule your pre-surgery exam several weeks in advance.

☐ Arrange for the help you will need during your recovery. If you will be at home, ask someone to stay with you for the first few days to a week. Make sure you have people to drive you to buy groceries, go to the doctor, etc.

☐ Schedule your pre-surgery exam anytime within 30 days of your surgery date.

☐ Call your insurance company to review your coverage for when you are in the hospital and when you leave.

☐ Go to the dentist, if you haven't gone within the last year.

☐ Eat a well-balanced, healthy diet.

☐ Start doing your strengthening exercises. (See page 20.)

☐ Write down any questions you have about your hospital stay and recovery. You can ask these at your pre-surgery exam. For questions about your surgery, call the surgeon's office.

3 weeks before surgery

☐ Get your home ready for your recovery. Make some meals that you can freeze and reheat later. Stock up on basic foods and easy-to-make meals.

☐ Have your pre-surgery exam and blood tests, if you haven't already. You need to do this within 30 days of your surgery.

☐ If you live alone and have a pet, arrange for someone to take care of the pet while you're in the hospital.

☐ Stop mail and newspaper delivery, unless someone will bring them in for you.

☐ Keep doing your strengthening exercises.

1 week before surgery

☐ Talk to your doctor about the medicines you take. Find out which ones you need to stop taking.

☐ Stop taking aspirin, ibuprofen and other anti-inflammatory drugs (such as Aleve). Tylenol is okay.

☐ Keep doing your strengthening exercises.

☐ Learn the breathing exercises you'll do after surgery. (See page 36.) Practice them every day.

1 day before surgery

☐ Pack the items you will bring with you to the hospital.

☐ Follow the rules your health care team gave you about diet and bathing.

☐ Make sure you have a ride to and from the hospital.

Tip

_____

Don't forget to arrange for a ride to and from the hospital.

Chapter 3

Getting Ready for Surgery

Before you have major surgery, you want to be in the best shape you can be. This means you should be in good health. If you have any sign of illness, severe heart or lung disease or other problems, your surgery may have to be postponed.

You will want to strengthen your upper-body and hip muscles before surgery. You should also learn your breathing exercises. All of this will help with your recovery.

Staying healthy

The better your overall health is, the less chance you are to have problems during or after surgery. To stay in good health:

- **Eat a healthy diet.** Good nutrition can help you heal and lower the chance of infection. A healthy diet includes plenty of fruits and vegetables and is low in fat and sugar. If you have questions or concerns about your diet, talk to a nurse or dietician.

- **Stop smoking.** If you quit smoking, even the week before surgery, it will lower your risks from surgery. You are not allowed to smoke in the hospital. If you need help quitting, tell your care team.

Tip

_____

See your dentist six weeks before surgery. If your gums or teeth get infected, you are more likely to get an infection in the hip.

- **Stay active.** Exercise improves your heart and lungs and boosts your immune system. But staying active when your hip hurts can be tough. Try swimming, water exercises and riding a stationary bike. These give you exercise without putting stress on your hip.

- **Take care of your teeth.** If you have not had a dental checkup within the last year, see your dentist at least six weeks before surgery. When teeth or gums become infected, bacteria (germs) can travel to the new hip joint. If the tissue around your new hip gets infected, you may need more surgery. It's best to have dental work done well before your hip is replaced.

Strengthening exercises

You may have become less active because of the pain and stiffness in your hip. When muscles are not used, they become weak. After you have your hip replaced, the joint problem will be fixed, but your muscles may still be weak. To make them stronger, you will follow a regular exercise program.

Start doing your exercises before your surgery. This way, it will be easier to do them after surgery. Getting stronger now will also speed your recovery.

Tip

_____

Start your exercises now. This will help you heal faster after surgery.

You will strengthen the muscles in your legs, buttocks and hips. These will support your new hip joint. It's also a good idea to strengthen your upper-body muscles. These will help you pull yourself up, sit up and push yourself around in bed. Strong arms also help you use crutches or a walker.

Practice the following exercises before your surgery. Most of these exercises are done lying down. You can do them in bed if you like. **Do not hold your breath while you exercise.**

Repeat each exercise 10 times or until your muscle feels tired. You are the best judge of how much you can do each day. If you feel pain, stop doing that exercise.

Ankle pumps and circles

For pumps, slowly flex your foot toward you, then away from you. For circles, move your foot around in circles, first in one direction, then the other.

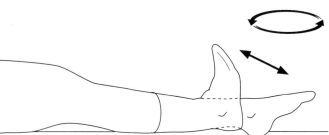

Thigh squeezes

Lying flat, press the back of your knee into the bed. At the same time, tighten your thigh. Hold for 5 seconds. Switch legs.

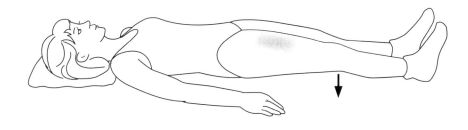

Buttocks squeezes

Tighten your buttocks muscles by squeezing them together. Hold for 5 seconds.

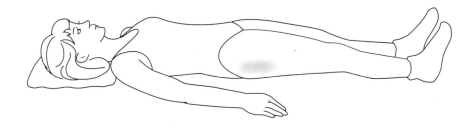

Hamstring sets

Slightly bend the knee on the side of your bad hip. Tighten the muscle at the back of your thigh (hamstring) by pressing your heel into the bed. Hold for 5 seconds.

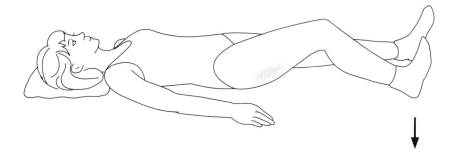

Heel slides

Slide your heel toward your buttocks, bending your knee. Keep your heel on the bed and your kneecap pointed to the ceiling.

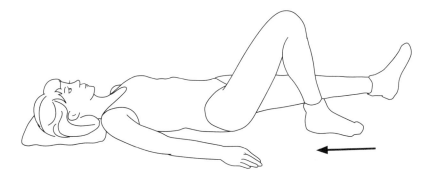

Lying kicks

Lie on your back. Place a rolled-up blanket under the knee of your sore leg. Straighten your knee, keeping the back of your thigh on the blanket the whole time. Hold for 5 seconds.

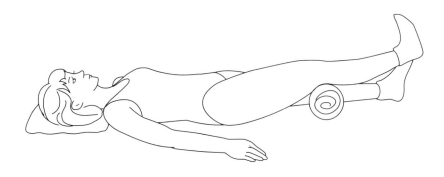

Sitting kicks

Sit in a sturdy chair. Straighten the knee of one leg as much as you can. Hold your leg up for 5 seconds. Switch legs.

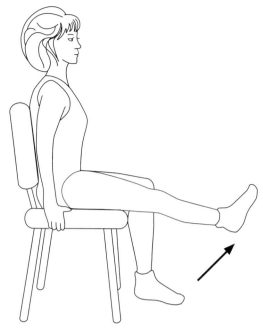

Bed sit-ups

Lie flat on your back. Come up on both elbows, then up on both hands. With your arms straight out behind you, come to a sitting position. Now reverse: lower yourself onto your elbows, then flat on your back.

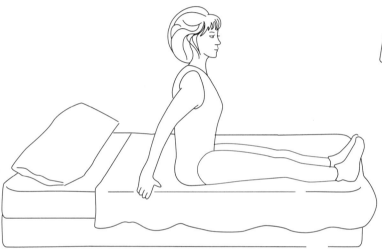

Chair push-ups

Sit in a sturdy chair with arms, or in a wheelchair with the wheels locked. Hold the chair arms. Push down on the chair arms and straighten your elbows. Push yourself up off the chair as much as you can, then slowly lower yourself back down.

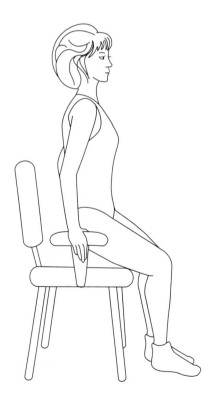

Straight leg raises

Lie flat on your back. With your knee straight, tighten your thigh muscle. As your thigh muscle tightens, lift your leg several inches off the bed. Keep your leg straight. Hold for 5 seconds, then slowly lower your leg.

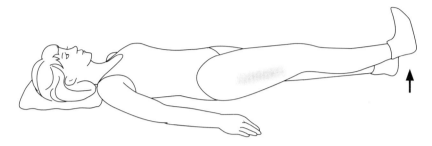

Leg slides

Lying on your back, slide your leg out to the side as far as you can. Keep your kneecap facing the ceiling. Then, bring your leg back. Repeat on both sides.

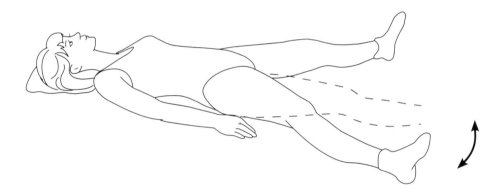

Side leg lifts

Lie on the side of your good hip. Lift your other leg as high as you can toward the ceiling. Keep the leg straight as you lift. Hold for 5 seconds, then slowly lower. Repeat on the other side if you're able.

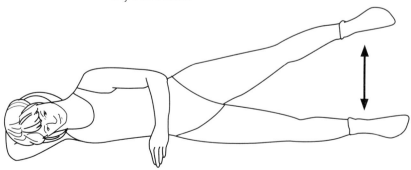

Breathing exercises

After surgery, you will be asked to do breathing exercises. These help prevent pneumonia and other lung problems. The exercises include deep breathing and coughing. It's a good idea to learn these exercises before surgery. Practice them every day for at least a week before you go in the hospital.

Deep breathing

Deep breathing helps fill your lungs completely. When you are doing it right, deep breathing uses your stomach muscles as well as your chest muscles.

1. Breathe in through your nose as deeply as you can. Hold for several seconds. Your stomach should go out as you breathe in.

2. Let your breath out through your mouth, slowly, so that all the breath goes out. Purse your lips as you let your breath out, like blowing out a candle. Your stomach should go in as you breathe out.

Breathe out for twice as long as you breathe in. Repeat 10 times.

Coughing

Coughing helps keep your lungs clear. Follow these steps.

1. Take a slow, deep breath. Breathe in through your nose. Focus on fully expanding your chest and back.

2. Breathe out through your mouth. Feel your chest sink downward and inward.

3. Take another breath in the same way.

4. Take a third breath. This time, hold your breath for a moment and then cough hard. As you cough, focus on forcing all the air out of your chest.

Repeat this exercise two more times.

Tip

If you practice your breathing exercises before surgery, they will be easier to do afterward—and you will be less likely to have lung problems.

Pre-surgery exam

You will see your doctor for a checkup within 30 days of your surgery. At this time you may have several tests, including blood tests. These tests give a good picture of your overall health.

Tip

Write down the name and dose of every medicine, herb and vitamin you take. Bring this list to your health exam.

During this exam, it's important to tell your doctor about all your medicines. Bring a written list of your medicines and the amounts you normally take. Also bring a list of past surgeries and hospital stays.

One week before surgery, you will need to stop taking aspirin and anti-inflammatory medicines. (These are drugs that reduce fever and swelling. They include Advil, Motrin, Aleve, Naprosyn, Feldene, Relafen, DayPro and others.) If you take these medicines every day for pain, ask your doctor how you can relieve pain during the week before surgery.

Your doctor will tell you if you need to stop any other medicines before surgery. Make sure you know:

- When to stop taking your medicines

- When to stop taking vitamins and herbal products (such as gingko, St. John's wort, garlic or echinacea)

- Which medicines you should take the morning of surgery, and how to take them (including diabetes medicines)

If you aren't sure if the drugs you take should be stopped, ask your doctor.

The day before surgery

- **Diet.** It's important to have an empty stomach before surgery. This will make the surgery as safe as possible. Your surgeon will tell you when to stop eating and drinking. If you don't follow his or her orders, your surgery could be changed to another date.

- **Bathing.** Your care team will tell you when and how to bathe before surgery. You will use anti-bacterial soap, such as Dial, or the special soap you get from your doctor. This soap helps kill germs and prevent infection.

- **Changes in health.** Call your doctor if there is any change in your health. Examples include a sore throat, runny nose, cough, fever, dental problems, urinating problems or skin problems, such as a rash, scrape or cut. These may mean that your surgery has to be postponed.

- **Other tips.** Do not smoke, drink alcohol or take over-the-counter medicine (unless your surgeon tells you to) for 24 hours before surgery.

If you have any questions about your surgery or how to get ready, call your health care team.

Tip

Be sure to follow the rules for eating and drinking before surgery. If you have any questions, call your surgeon's office.

Chapter 4

Your Hospital Stay

Your care team will tell you what to expect at the hospital.

Before surgery

After checking in at the hospital, you will be asked to sign one or more consent forms. These forms state that you know the risks and benefits of surgery. When you sign the forms, you give your care team permission to do the surgery. Do not sign them unless you understand what will happen during and after your surgery.

Next you will go to the pre-surgery area, where you will be "prepped" (prepared) for surgery. Friends and family can stay with you there. When you're in surgery, they will be in the waiting area.

Anesthesia

An anesthesia provider will talk with you about what kind of anesthesia (medicine) will be used. This medicine will keep you comfortable during surgery. The provider will check your health status and answer any questions you have about the medicine.

You will have either general or regional anesthesia. The choice depends on the type of surgery you're having, your health history and your current health.

With **general anesthesia** you are asleep during surgery. You may receive the medicine through your IV tube or breathe it in through your nose. During surgery, a breathing tube helps you breathe while you are asleep. Afterward, you may feel some minor side effects, such as a sore throat, headache, hoarse voice, feeling sick to your stomach and feeling sleepy.

Regional anesthesia will make you lose all feeling from your lower back to your toes. You may receive this medicine through a shot in your lower back (called spinal anesthesia). It does not put you to sleep, but you may remember very little about the surgery. This is due to other medicines you may receive through your IV line. The most common side effects are small headaches that last for a few days and trouble passing urine when using the toilet.

After surgery

Surgery often takes from one to four hours. With the "prep" time and wake-up time, you'll be in the operating room and recovery room for several hours.

It could take one to three hours for your anesthesia to wear off. In the recovery room, nurses will check your blood pressure, pulse and breathing. They will help you with any side effects from the anesthesia.

When you wake up:

- You may have an oxygen mask.

- You might have blurred vision and a dry mouth.

- You may feel sick to your stomach. If you vomit (throw up) or feel sick, you may receive medicine to help you feel better.

- You may be confused, drowsy and dizzy. Don't try to get up alone—you may be weaker than you think. Your nurse will help you when you first try to walk.

- You may feel some pain. Your nurse will make you as comfortable as possible. He or she will ask you to rate your pain using a pain scale. This tells your care team how much pain medicine to give you. If you had spinal anesthesia, you might not feel any pain right after surgery.

- A large bandage will cover the surgical area to keep it clean.

- You may have tubes that drain fluid from the surgical wound. (This is called an incision drain.) The fluid goes into a special container. Your care team will keep track of the amount of fluid that comes out.

- You'll receive fluids and medicines through an IV line in your arm.

- You may have a tube (catheter) in your bladder to remove urine.

When you are fully awake, you will be moved to your hospital room. Your family and friends can visit you there. You might have a room to yourself, or you may share a room with another patient.

Dealing with pain

As your body heals, you might feel a stabbing, pinching or aching pain. Treating pain is an important part of your care.

Tell your health care team about any pain you feel. Remember, all pain is real. You have the right to have it treated.

Your pain can be affected by how you feel about other things in your life. For example, worries about your job, money or family can cause stress and make your pain worse. Share your worries with your health care team. They can help you deal with the issues that add to your stress and pain.

Pain scale

Everyone feels pain in a different way. You may be asked to rate your pain using a pain scale. (For example, you might rate your pain on a scale from 1 to 10.) This will help your care team know how much pain you feel.

Tell your health care team:

*   Where you feel pain and how much pain you have

*   What makes your pain better or worse

*   Which pain medicines have worked for you in the past

There are many ways to relieve pain. Your care team can help you decide what works best for you. The right treatment will make you more comfortable so you can get back to your normal routine. When your pain is under control, you will be better able to heal. Your pain will get better each day.

Tip
_____

As you wake up from surgery, tell your nurse if:

*   *You need pain medicine.*

*   *You feel sick to your stomach.*

*   *Your legs or feet hurt, tingle or feel numb.*

Pain medicine

After surgery you will receive medicine for your pain. For severe pain, you may receive strong medicines called narcotics. (Morphine, Dilaudid and codeine are examples of narcotics.) They work well, but they might make you drowsy, itchy or sick to your stomach. If you take narcotics, try to take the pills with food.

For mild or medium pain, you may receive drugs to reduce swelling and soreness (such as Tylenol, aspirin and ibuprofen). These may be used along with narcotics. They can have side effects, too, such as making you sick to your stomach.

There are different ways to take pain medicine. Depending on your doctor's orders, you may have medicine as a pill, as a shot or in your IV line.

After surgery, you may have a button you can push to control your pain yourself. This will pump pain medicine through your IV and into your body. The pump is set so you cannot give yourself too much medicine at one time. **Only you can touch this button. Family and other visitors may not touch this button.**

Here are some tips for taking pain medicine:

- Ask for medicine when you need it. Don't try to "tough it out"—this can make you feel worse. It's rare to get addicted to the kind of pain medicine used after surgery.

- Take your medicine as soon as you feel pain. Don't wait for pain to get worse before taking medicine.

- Medicine doesn't work the same for everyone. If yours isn't working, tell your nurse. He or she can try other medicines.

- Take pain medicine at least 45 minutes before physical therapy or other activities.

Your care team will watch for side effects from the medicines. If you feel sick, "off" or uncomfortable after taking medicine, tell your nurse.

Keep in mind that medicine won't take away all of your pain. It helps to try other ways to relax and ease pain.

Tip

Tell your nurse if you feel sick after taking medicine, or if you just don't feel right. Your doctor may order a different medicine for you.

Ice, massage and movement

Ice packs, self-massage and moving your body into a different position all can help with pain. You may ask your nurse for ice or for a cold pack.

Relaxation

You can use your mind to reduce pain.

- **Visualize.** Imagine yourself in a nice place where you feel good. This might be at a beach, in a park or at home on your couch.

- **Distract yourself.** Do something to take your mind off the pain. For example, talk with a friend or play a game.

- **Listen to music.** For many people, calming music helps them feel better.

- **Breathe slowly.** If you focus on your breathing and let other thoughts go out of your mind, your pain may slip away for a while.

Visitors at the Hospital

During the first few days after surgery, you will be busy learning to use your new hip. You will need plenty of rest. Your care team will help you balance active times with rest periods.

The support of family and friends will help your recovery. But having too many visitors can take away from the rest you need. You may prefer to limit your visitors. Ask some people to save their visits until you are home.

Starting your recovery

Care equipment

Your care team may use special equipment to help you heal.

- **Abductor pillow.** This is a triangle-shaped pillow. It fits between your legs to keep them from crossing when you are in bed.

- **Breathing device (incentive spirometer).** This helps you do your deep breathing exercises in the first few days after surgery.

- **Elastic stockings.** These tight-fitting socks, known as TED stockings, may help prevent blood clots in your legs after surgery.

Activity

At first you may not feel like doing anything at all, but movement and exercise are crucial to recovery. Soon you will begin doing exercises with the help of your physical therapist and nurses. But for now, remember:

- It's important to follow guidelines on how to use your hip safely. These are found on pages 40 to 42.

- If you want to get out of bed, ask for help. **Do not get out of bed by yourself.**

- Ask your nurse how far you may raise the head of your bed. Sitting up too high may cause the ball of your hip to come out of its socket (dislocation).

- Some people have a sore back after surgery. Changing positions in bed once in a while will help.

Diet

Your diet may start with ice chips and liquids. You will begin eating regular meals as your body is able—when your stomach growls and you can pass gas. Tell your nurse if you'd like to meet with a dietician.

Tip

Do not get out of bed by yourself. Press the call button, and a nurse will come help you.

After your IV line is taken out, try to drink six to eight glasses of water each day. Drinking plenty of fluids helps prevent constipation (hard stools). Tell your nurse if you feel sick to your stomach and can't drink water.

Breathing exercises

Right after surgery, you will start your breathing exercises—deep breathing, coughing and using your breathing device. These help to keep your lungs clear and prevent problems like pneumonia.

Therapy

Therapy is very important to your recovery.

- **Physical therapy** teaches you how to move your hip safely, so that your new hip joint does not move out of place. It also helps you to strengthen the muscles around your new hip.

- **Occupational therapy** teaches you how to safely do everyday activities, such as bathing, getting dressed, cooking and cleaning. The therapist may suggest some equipment to make these tasks easier.

You will begin therapy soon after your surgery. You can start with ankle pumps and circles while you're lying in bed. The day after your operation, a nurse or physical therapist will help you stand up and sit in a chair. You may begin walking with help. You will be shown how to safely move your legs and hips and how to use a walker or crutches.

Each day of your hospital stay, you will do more exercises and walk a little more. Over time, you will put more and more weight on your new hip.

Before you leave the hospital, you will learn a set of exercises to do at home.

Tip

Take your pain medicine 45 minutes before therapy.

Care plan

Your care plan describes what will happen while you are in the hospital. It helps you understand your treatment and the goals you and your health care team will work on before you go home. Your care plan may change depending on your needs. Feel free to ask questions of your care team during your hospital stay.

You will heal faster if you do as much as you can for yourself throughout your hospital stay. Your nurses will advise you on what you can do. Each day your physical activity should increase.

It's also important to express your feelings and concerns. Talk with your family or friends about what you might need after you leave the hospital.

Your goals

During your hospital stay, you'll work toward a number of goals with the help of your care team. Before you go home, you should be able to:

- Get safely in and out of bed, a chair and a car by yourself (or with a little help from your caregiver).

- Safely complete self-care activities, such as dressing and using the toilet. (You may use help or equipment as needed).

- Walk safely with a walker or crutches.

- Begin your home exercise program.

- Follow guidelines for hip safety.

- Know how to manage your pain.

- Know the signs of infection.

- Go to the bathroom (urinate and move your bowels) as you did before your hospital stay.

- Eat a well-balanced diet to promote healing.

- Feel sure that you or your caregiver can meet your needs.

Tip

Try to do things for yourself when you're in the hospital. This will help you heal faster.

Each day of your hospital stay

Tip
_____

Tell your nurse how you
feel. He or she can give
you medicine if you have
pain or nausea (feel sick
to your stomach).

- The nurse will check your blood pressure, pulse, temperature and breathing. He or she will also check the feeling, movement and color of your legs and feet. Your lungs and abdomen will be checked as well.

- If you feel pain or sick to your stomach, ask your nurse for medicine. You may be asked to rate your level of pain. Ask for pain medicine at least 45 minutes before doing any major activity or physical therapy.

- You may receive medicine to prevent blood clots. To make sure the medicine is working, you may be given blood tests.

- Your nurse will urge you to cough, take deep breaths and use your breathing device every 1 to 2 hours while you're awake.

- You will have physical therapy.

- A pillow will be used to keep your legs apart in bed.

- You'll wear elastic stockings to prevent blood clots in your legs. The stockings may be removed two to three times a day.

- Do ankle pumps 10 times an hour. (See page 21.) This improves blood flow in your legs.

- Remember your hip safety. (See pages 40 to 42.)

First day after surgery

- Your nurse or therapist will help you stand up and sit in a chair. You may begin walking and exercising with help.

- You may begin pain pills.

- You may start eating regular foods.

- You may receive fluids, medicine and blood through an IV line in your arm.

- Your care team may remove your incision drain.

- Your nurse may change the bandage over the surgical area.

Second day after surgery

- You will walk and exercise at least two times with your physical therapist and nurses.

- Your care team may remove your IV and bladder tubes. They may also remove your incision drain if they have not yet done so.

- Your nurse will change your bandages as needed.

- Talk with your nurse about your normal bathroom habits. If you do not have a bowel movement today, you may need a laxative (medicine to help you go to the bathroom).

- You will start occupational therapy.

Third day after surgery/Last day in the hospital

- Continue to increase your walking distance and leg strength.

- Make final plans for after your hospital stay. A social worker or care coordinator can help.

- Your physical therapist will teach you how to get in and out of a car and climb stairs. The therapist will also show you a home exercise program. Please bring this book to your physical therapy session.

- Ask a family member or your caregiver to come to a therapy session.

- Ask a family member to bring your walker or crutches to the hospital.

Tip

Bring this book with you to therapy sessions. It's a good idea to bring a family member or friend, too.

Hip safety

After hip replacement surgery, one of the first things you may notice is relief from the constant pain you had in your hip. That alone may make you want to get up and dance. But you need to be careful about how you use your new hip at first. To protect your hip, you must limit some of your movements.

Follow these safety rules:

• Don't bend your hips more than your doctor says.

• Keep your legs apart.

• Keep your toes pointed up, not to the side, when lying down.

Do's and don't's

Do:

- Keep knees shoulder-width apart.

- Keep your operated leg facing forward when sitting or walking.

- Keep your operated leg in front while getting up.

- Keep your toes pointed up, not to the side, when lying down.

- Keep your knee no higher than your operated hip when sitting.

- Sit up straight, but **do not** lean forward.

- Grasp chair arms to help you get up safely.

- Use a foam pillow between your legs while sleeping.

- Keep a pillow between your legs when you roll onto your "good" side.

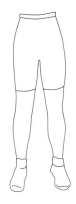

Keep knees shoulder-width apart, with toes pointing forward.

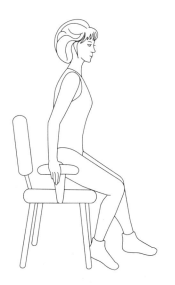

Keep your sore leg in front when getting up from a chair. Grasp the chair arms to help you get up safely.

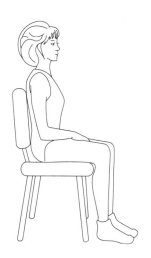

Sit up straight, but do not lean forward. Your knee should never be higher than your hip.

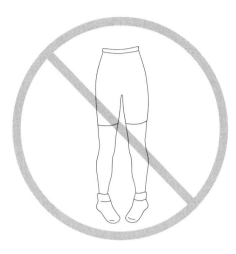

Don't turn your leg inward or outward. Don't cross your legs or ankles.

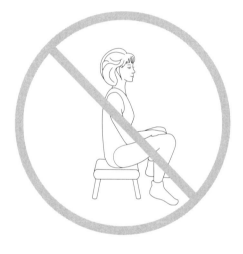

Don't sit on a low chair. Always keep your knee lower than your hip.

Don't:

- Don't cross your legs or ankles.

- Don't turn your leg or kneecap inward or outward when sitting, standing or lying down. Your feet should never point toward or away from each other.

- Don't bring your knee toward your chest.

- Don't bend your hips more than your doctor tells you. For example, don't bend over to pick things up from the floor or reach in a low cupboard.

- Don't use your hand, your strong leg or anything else to force your operated hip to move.

- Don't sit up in bed with your knees bent.

- Don't lean forward in bed to pull up your blankets.

- Don't sit and twist to reach objects.

- Don't twist or pivot on your operated leg.

- Don't sit in a low, soft chair or sofa. Don't sit on a low toilet or stool.

- Don't drive until your doctor says it's okay.

- Don't reach for objects by turning your shoulders without also turning your pelvis.

- Don't swing your operated leg behind you, unless your doctor says it's okay.

Don't turn your shoulders without also turning your pelvis.

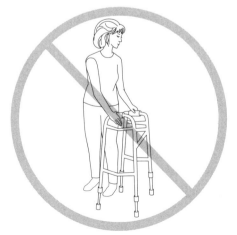

Getting ready to leave the hospital

Your care team will let you know when you can leave the hospital. Before you leave, they will review guidelines for:

- Hip safety

- Preventing falls

- Wound care

- Nutrition

- Problems to watch for

- Activity level

- Home exercises

- Equipment

- Bathing

- Elastic stockings

- Medicines

- Follow-up visits

These guidelines are covered in the next chapter. If you have any questions, ask your doctor or nurse.

Preventing Complications

Every surgery has its risks. With hip replacement surgery, the major risks include blood clots, infection, the joint popping out of place (dislocation) and loosening of the joint.

While you are in the hospital, your care team will take many steps to prevent these problems. For example:

- They will take your blood pressure, temperature and pulse often.

- They will check the movement, feeling, circulation and pulse in your leg.

- You will do exercises that improve circulation and strength.

- You will wear TED stockings (elastic socks) to help prevent blood clots.

- Your care team will give you medicine to help keep blood clots from forming.

- You will do breathing exercises to keep your lungs clear and healthy.

- Your care team will check your bandage and surgical wound often. Tubes will drain extra blood and fluid away from the wound area.

- A physical therapist will show you how to move your hip safely. Following the safety guidelines will help keep the new joint in place.

Some problems do not show up until long after surgery. Before you leave the hospital, you will learn what problems to watch for (see page 65).

Chapter 5

Living with Your New Hip

By the time you leave the hospital, you should be able to do some things on your own, such as walk with crutches or a walker, get in and out of a bed or chair, and climb a few stairs.

Before you leave, you will be given advice and rules to follow. These rules help make your recovery safe and smooth. If you have any questions, be sure to ask your care team.

You will need someone to drive you home or to another care facility. Your social worker or care coordinator can arrange transportation if you need it.

What happens when you go home

Recovery takes time. Most people get back to their normal routine in six to eight weeks. Many use a walker or crutches for four to six weeks, then use a cane for another month or so. For some, progress is quicker.

Full recovery can take three to six months, depending on your health and how well you do with therapy.

Medicines

When you get home, you'll keep taking the medicines your doctor prescribed. These might include drugs to prevent blood clots, such as Coumadin (warfarin) or aspirin. Another drug to prevent blood clots is heparin (Enoxaparin). This is taken as a shot. Your care team will teach you or a family member how to give a shot if you are taking this medicine.

Your doctor will also prescribe pain pills. These can make your therapy and hip exercises more comfortable. Take your pain medicine 45 minutes before you exercise—it's easier to prevent pain than to treat it after it's started. Let your care team know if you have trouble controlling pain. Most people stop needing pain medicine after a few weeks.

Some people also take medicine to help with sleep or to relax their muscles.

Wound care

You must keep the area around your incision (cut) clean while it heals. You will need someone to help you care for the wound.

- Look at it every day. Call your doctor if you see any redness, swelling or fluid draining from it, or if it feels warm or more painful.

- Change your bandage the way your care team showed you. Do not use any cream or ointment on the wound.

- If Steri-Strips (strips of tape) were used on the cut, they will fall off as it heals. You don't need to replace them.

- If staples were used, they will be removed at your next doctor visit or by a home health aide.

- If a clear suture (a stitch that looks like a fishing line) is sticking out from your incision, cut it flush with the skin. The rest of the suture will dissolve.

Few people are pain-free when they leave the hospital. Expect to take pain killers for the first couple weeks.

Elastic socks

Keep wearing the white elastic stockings (TEDs) you got at the hospital. You should wear them until your first doctor visit after the surgery.

You can take the socks off twice a day for 15 minutes—ask someone to help you. It's fine to wash and dry them before you put them back on.

Eating

When you leave the hospital, go back to your normal diet as soon as you can. Do not skip meals. Eat breakfast, lunch and dinner.

A well-balanced diet will help you feel good and recover quickly. Choose a range of fruits, vegetables, grains, milk products and meat. It's also important to drink plenty of fluids.

Be sure to include:

- **High-fiber foods.** Fiber helps keep your bowel movements regular and prevents constipation (hard stools). Good sources of fiber include whole grains, brown rice, cracked wheat (bulgur), oatmeal, popcorn, whole oats, rye and wheat. Fruits and vegetables are also great sources of fiber—plus they are low in fat and packed with nutrients.

- **High-calcium foods.** Calcium helps build strong bones. Good sources of calcium include milk, yogurt, cheese, enriched soymilk, tofu, soups made with milk, and dark green, leafy vegetables (such as kale or collard greens). Choose low-fat or fat-free dairy products. If you don't eat milk products, eat other foods that contain calcium. Ask your doctor if a calcium pill is a good idea for you.

- **Iron-rich foods.** This mineral helps your blood carry oxygen to every part of your body. Good sources of iron include lean meats, dark turkey meat, shellfish (such as shrimp), cooked dry beans or peas and whole grain breads.

If you have concerns about your eating plan, ask your nurse about setting up a visit with a dietician.

Tip

Be sure to drink lots of water and other fluids. This will help prevent constipation (hard stools).

Questions and Answers about Recovery

How long will I need to follow the hip safety rules?

Most people need to do this for at least six to 12 weeks. Your doctor will tell you more at your follow-up visit.

How long will I be in pain?

As your muscles and tissues heal, the pain you feel in your hip will get better. Most of the pain should go away in about a month. After that, it's normal to feel some aches once in a while, but severe pain is not normal.

When can I drive?

Your doctor will let you know when you can drive. Many surgeons advise against driving for at least six weeks after surgery. Do not drive while taking pain pills, because they can make your driving unsafe.

How soon can I take a bath or shower?

Your care team will let you know when you can take a shower or bath. You may have to wait several weeks before you can soak in the tub.

How long do I have to use the abductor pillow?

Use this for six weeks or until your doctor tells you to stop.

Will my new hip joint set off alarms at the airport?

Yes. When it does, tell the airport workers that you have an artificial hip. They will do a security check on you before you board the plane.

Questions and Answers about Recovery

What if I'm constipated?

Many people have constipation (hard stools) after hip surgery. This is often caused by pain medicine, being less active and taking iron pills.

To help prevent constipation:

- Drink eight to 10 glasses of fluid each day.

- Stay active.

- Eat more fiber. Choose whole-grain breads, bran cereals and fresh fruits and vegetables.

- Stop using pain pills when you can.

If you have trouble with constipation, talk to your care team. They may suggest that you take a stool softener, laxative or other medicine to relieve the problem.

When can I have sex?

Ask your doctor. For most people, it's fine to have sex about four to six weeks after surgery. This allows time for the wound and muscles to heal.

When you become sexually active again, use a firm mattress. Many people, men and women, find it easier to lie on their back during sex. This position takes less energy and lowers the chance of dislocation.

What is a hip dislocation? Are there any warning signs?

A dislocation is when the ball of the hip joint slips out of the socket. To prevent this, follow the hip safety rules on pages 40 to 42.

If the hip does pop out, it will happen in a fraction of a second, without warning. You will feel severe pain in your groin and be unable to move your new hip fully. **If this happens to you, call 911.**

Bathing

You will be told when you can shower and get your wound wet. Do not soak in a bathtub until your doctor says it's okay.

If you have staples or stitches, cover them with plastic to keep the wound dry when you're taking a shower. Use a tub or shower chair for support until you can get around more easily. (See page 60.) Tips on getting in and out of the tub are found on page 55.

Therapy

You may still have physical therapy at the hospital or at home. Your care team will tell you how long you may need therapy.

The therapist will review your hip safety guidelines and help you with the exercises you'll do at home. You might also work on balance, safe walking and muscle strength. An occupational therapist may help you with day-to-day tasks.

Movement and activity

After surgery, most people feel less pain than they have in a long time. You may find yourself able to do things you have avoided.

Tip

_____

For at least six weeks after surgery, use a pillow between your legs while sleeping.

Walking and other light activities will help you regain the use of your hip joint and muscles. Still, you need to use your hip in safe ways until it heals. Follow the hip safety rules on pages 40 to 42.

You also need to be careful when doing everyday tasks like getting out of bed, going up and down stairs, cooking and cleaning. The following are tips about how to do daily tasks without hurting your hip. As a general rule, avoid movements or positions that cause pain or discomfort in your hip.

Getting in and out of bed

To get into bed:

- Back up toward the bed until you feel it against your legs. Place your operated leg forward.

- Reaching back with one hand at a time, slowly lower yourself onto the edge of the bed.

- Scoot back until your thighs are supported by the edge of the bed.

- Support your upper body with your arms, then bring your legs into the bed. To lift your operated leg, you may need to use a crutch, cane, belt or leg lifter (see page 58). Or, ask someone for help.

- Keep your body in a straight line with your legs. Do not cross, twist or bend your legs.

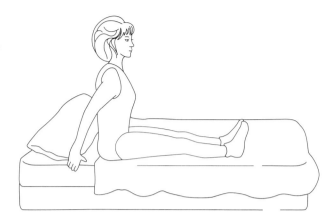

Do not bend your knees or cross your legs when getting in or out of bed. Keep you body and legs in a straight line.

To get out of bed:

- Come to a sitting position in the bed. Do not bend your knees.

- Turn your body and move your legs off the bed. To move your leg, you may need to use a crutch, cane, belt or leg lifter (see page 58). Or, ask someone for help.

- Keep your body in a straight line with your legs. Move to sit at the edge of the bed.

- Place your operated leg forward.

- Push off the bed and stand up.

Using a walker or crutches

Use a walker or crutches until your care team tells you to stop. Your doctor will let you know how much weight you can place on your leg.

To walk:

- Stand up straight, with your weight evenly balanced on the walker or crutches. Keep the walker flat on the floor.

- Move the walker or crutches forward a little. Then, step forward. Lift your operated leg so that the heel of your foot touches the floor first.

- Try to walk as smoothly as you can. Over time you will put more and more weight on your leg.

- Do not turn too quickly. Take small steps and turn toward your strong leg.

To sit:

- Back up until you feel the chair against the back of your legs.

- Slide your operated leg forward, then lower yourself slowly into the chair. Use the armrests.

To stand:

- Come to the edge of the chair with your operated leg out in front of you.

- Use both arms to push yourself up to standing, then reach for your walker.

- Do not use the walker to pull yourself up.

Tip

Never use your walker to pull yourself up from a seated position.

From Walker to Cane

Many people use a walker for the first several weeks after hip surgery. A walker helps with balance and keeps you from falling. After that, you may use a cane or single crutch for several more weeks until you get your strength and balance back.

You are ready to use a cane or single crutch when:

- You can stand and balance without your walker.

- Your weight is placed fully on both feet.

- You no longer lean on your hands when using your walker.

Carry your cane or crutch in the hand opposite your sore hip. For example, if you had surgery on your left hip, use the cane with your right hand.

Using the toilet

You will need to use a toilet with a raised seat. (See page 58.)

- To sit down, back up to the toilet until you can feel it against your legs.

- Move your operated leg forward. Reach back with both hands and grab the safety rails, armrests or raised toilet seat.

- Slowly lower yourself onto the toilet, using both arms.

- To stand up, slide to the edge of the toilet and move your operated leg forward. Place both hands behind you on the toilet seat.

- Push off with both arms to raise yourself off the toilet.

- When your balance is steady, reach for your walker or crutches. Never try to pull yourself up from the toilet by grabbing your walker.

Sitting and standing

It's best to sit in a firm chair with arms. That way you can push off with your arms to stand up. Do not sit in a low or over-stuffed chair or couch. You have to bend your hips too much to get up again.

Tip

_____

Do not sit for more than one hour at a time. (This includes riding in a car.) Get up and stretch or walk a little. When you're sitting, remember to keep your knees and legs apart.

If you need to use an armless chair, follow these steps:

- Approach the chair from the side.

- Slide your operated leg in front of you.

- Holding the edge of the seat and the back of the chair, slowly sit down. Then turn to face forward in the chair.

- To stand up, turn your body so you are sitting sideways in the chair.

- Slide your operated leg in front of you.

- Push up from the chair with both hands. Place one hand on the back of the chair.

- When your balance is steady, reach for your walker or crutches.

Bathing

Until your stitches or staples are removed, you will need to take sponge baths. Ask your doctor when it is safe for you to take a shower.

When you start taking baths and showers, it's a good idea to have handrails or grab bars in the tub. These will help with your balance and support. You can also use a long-handled sponge and a hand-held showerhead. If you use a bathtub, you will sit in a tub chair with your leg straight. The heel should rest on the edge of the tub.

Your occupational therapist can give you tips to make bathing easier. The first few times you take a bath or shower, have some-one nearby in case you need help.

To bathe or shower:

- Use a tub chair in the bathtub or shower. Do not sit on the floor of the bathtub.

- Back up to the tub chair and place your operated leg forward.

- Reach with one hand to the back of the tub seat or handrail. Reach the other hand to the front edge of the tub seat. Then, slowly turn and sit. Keep both hands on the tub seat or handrail while you lower yourself.

- Lift one leg into the tub at a time. Use a cane, crutch, belt or leg lifter to lift your operated leg. Or, ask someone to help you.

- To get out of the tub, use a cane, crutch or belt to lift your operated leg.

- Push up from the chair with both hands, or use the handrails to pull yourself up.

- When your balance is steady, reach for your walker or crutches.

Getting dressed

- Use your reacher to put on underwear and pants. (See page 58.)

- Do not lean forward to put your clothes on or tie your shoes.

- Use a sock aid to put on your socks. (See page 59.) Ask someone to help you if you can't do it yourself.

- Wear slip-on shoes or shoes with elastic laces. (See page 59.) These are easier to put on.

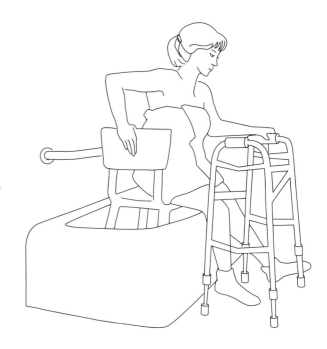

Use a tub chair to get in or out of the bathtub or shower.

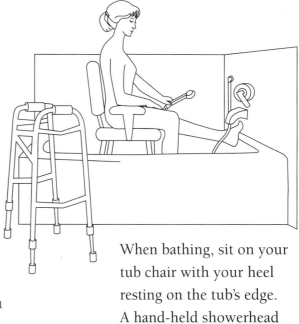

When bathing, sit on your tub chair with your heel resting on the tub's edge. A hand-held showerhead makes bathing easier.

Reaching, bending and carrying

You will need some help with laundry, cleaning and shopping when you get home. When you start doing housework, follow these tips:

- Use a long-handled reacher to turn on lights or grab things that are beyond arm's length. (See page 58.) Do not bend to reach in low cupboards.

- Do not carry or hold things in your hands while using a walker or crutches. Instead, carry things in an apron, pocket, fanny pack, backpack or walker basket.

- Do not reach too far when sliding items across a counter.

- Do not stand on tiptoes or chairs to reach high cupboards or storage areas.

- Use a rolling cart to carry hot, heavy or fragile items.

- Use a high stool (without wheels) when you cook or do dishes.

Going up and down stairs

- Remember: "up with the good" and "down with the bad." Go up the step with your good leg first. Then bring your other leg up to the same step. Go down with your "bad" leg first. Then bring your good leg down to the same step.

- Use the handrails for support.

- Do not try to climb steps that are higher than the standard height (7 inches).

Tip

Use equipment—a long-handled reacher, a walker basket, a rolling cart—to make your tasks easier.

Getting in and out of a car

Move your car seat back as far as it goes to increase the legroom. When you are getting in or out of the car, have the driver park away from the curb and not on a hill.

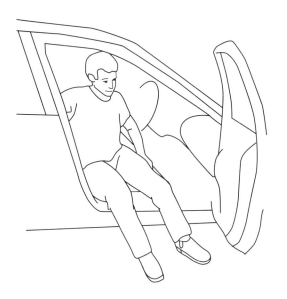

To get into a car:

- Back up to the front seat until you feel it at the back of your legs. Slide your operated leg forward.

- Reach back and find a stable place to hold onto, such as the dashboard and back of the seat. Slowly lower yourself onto the seat without twisting your body.

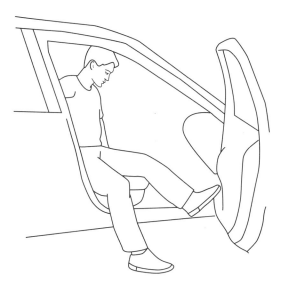

- Scoot back onto the seat. Keeping you body in line with your legs, slowly turn your body and lift your legs into the car so you are facing forward. Ask someone to help you lift your operated leg, or use a cane or crutch to lift it yourself.

- A plastic bag on the car seat may help you move more easily.

To get out of a car:

- Slowly turn your body as you move your legs out of the car. Keep your body in line with your legs. Use a cane or crutch to lift your operated leg, or ask someone else to do it.

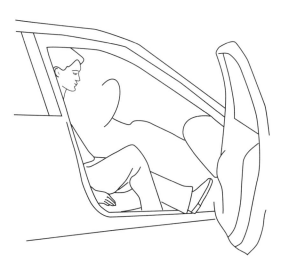

- Scoot to the edge of the seat and put your feet on the street (not the curb).

- Push with your arms and use your good leg to stand.

- When your balance is steady, reach for your walker or crutches.

Equipment that can help

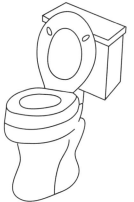

You can buy or rent special equipment to make tasks easier. You will need to use a walking aid—a walker, crutches or a cane. Your health care team may also want you to use a leg lifter, a raised toilet seat and a reacher. You may need other items as well.

The occupational therapist will show you how to get and use your equipment before you leave the hospital. (See "Where to get health equipment," page 61, and Resources, pages 69 to 70.)

Health insurance may cover only the cost of a walking aid. Call your insurance company to find out if anything else is covered.

Walking aids

A walker, crutches or a cane will help you walk after surgery.

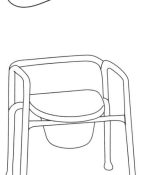

Raised toilet seat

This makes it easier for you to get on and off the toilet.

Commode

A portable toilet allows you to stay on one floor of your home if you don't have a bathroom on each level.

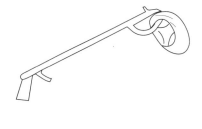

Reacher

A reacher helps you grab things that are too high or low. It can also help you put clothes on.

Leg lifter

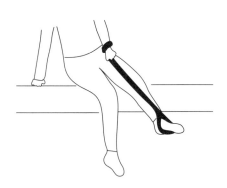

Use a leg lifter to move your operated leg safely in and out of a bed, car or bathtub.

Long-handled sponge

Use this to wash your feet, legs and back without bending.

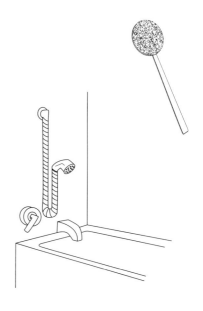

Hand-held showerhead

This lets you control the spray of water while sitting down in a tub or shower.

Elastic laces

Elastic laces allow you to put on shoes that are already tied.

Long-handled shoehorn

With the shoehorn, you can put your foot into a shoe without bending.

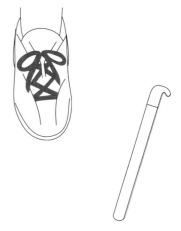

Sock aid

A sock aid helps you put on socks without bending.

Grab bars

Install grab bars to hold onto when getting on or off the toilet and in or out of the tub or shower.

Toilet tongs

Tongs allow you to use toilet paper without twisting your body.

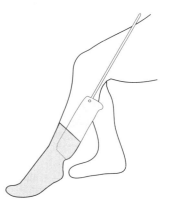

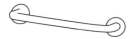

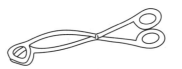

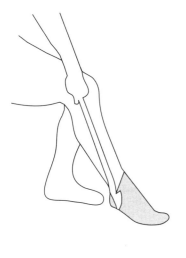

Dressing stick

You can use a dressing stick to get dressed without bending. To remove socks, slide the dressing stick down into the sock, by the heel. Push the sock off. To put on pants:

1. Hook the stick in the pants belt loop at the front of the leg you are dressing first, near the zipper.

2. Lower the pants to the floor and put your foot in.

3. Use the stick to pull the pants up to where you can reach them with your hand.

4. Repeat with the other leg.

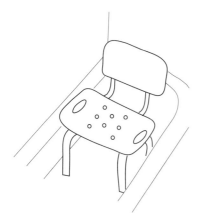

Tub or shower chair

This is useful if you can't stand up long enough to shower, or if you have trouble getting in or out of the tub. It is often used with a hand-held showerhead.

Tub transfer bench

A bench keeps you from stepping over the edge of the bathtub. It is useful for people who cannot bear full weight on their leg (who have a "weight-bearing restriction"). To use the bench:

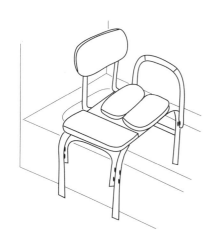

1. Come to the edge of the tub and turn around so you feel the bench at the back of your knees.

2. Lower yourself onto the bench and turn toward the tub.

3. Lift your feet over the edge of the tub one at a time while keeping your leg straight. Do not lift your knee higher than your hip.

4. To get out of the tub, use the same process in reverse.

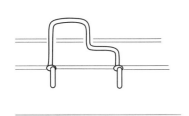

Clamp-on tub rail

You can hold onto this when getting in and out of the bathtub. This must be installed on the edge of your tub.

Where to Get Health Care Equipment

To find the items you need, try these ideas:

- Borrow them from friends or family.

- Call your local American Legion, VFW or Lions Club. They often have health care equipment that you can borrow.

- Call your local drugstore to see what items the store carries.

- Your care team may have mail-order catalogs that sell a range of equipment.

- Look in the Yellow Pages under "disabled persons' assistance" or "home health services" for agencies that sell equipment.

Work and hobbies

Ask your doctor when you can go back to work. If you have a desk job, you may be able to return to work fairly soon. It may take longer to go back to jobs that involve driving, walking or standing.

Many hobbies are fine to do soon after surgery. They are a good way to pass the time as you're recovering. But if your hobby involves heavy lifting or activity, hold off. Talk to your doctor if you are unsure about your activity level.

Exercise

Exercise can help prevent problems after surgery. It also builds your strength so you can get back to your normal routine.

Your leg muscles probably feel weak because you did not use them much when your hip was giving you trouble. After the surgery, regular exercise will help strengthen your weak muscles. The hip exercises you learned will make your hip stronger, allowing it to move smoothly and without pain.

Exercise also helps prevent constipation (hard stools). It keeps your joints flexible (able to move easily), improves muscle tone and makes you feel good. Without it, you will be weak and stiff.

Hip exercises

Your physical therapist will show you what exercises to do at home and how to do them correctly. Do these exercises two times a day for at least three months.

It's most comfortable to do the exercises lying down. Your bed is a good place. Don't lie on the floor.

It's normal to feel a little sore after exercise. But if you feel a lot of pain or muscle aches, talk to your care team.

Walking

Besides your home exercise program, make time each day for walking. Walking is a good form of physical therapy and makes your leg muscles stronger. It also builds your endurance. This means you'll be able to do more without feeling as tired.

Start by walking around your home several times each day. Trips to the bathroom or kitchen are not enough. Keep using your walker or crutches until your doctor tells you to stop. Later you can use a cane until you are steady enough to walk without one.

Work your way up to walking outdoors. At first, walk for 5 to 10 minutes a few times a day. As you become stronger, you may be able to walk for 20 to 30 minutes. After you have fully recovered, regular walks will help keep you strong.

Staying active

Some sports, such as basketball and running, are not good choices after hip replacement. But over time, most people are able to enjoy lighter activities, including golf, dancing and riding a bike.

Good choices for staying active include:

• Swimming

• Walking

• Water aerobics

• Riding a bike or stationary cycle

• Golf

• Dancing

• Cross-country skiing

These help you stay fit without too much wear on your new joint. But some activities will increase the risk of problems with your new hip.

Avoid these unless you have your doctor's approval:

Tip
_____

*When you exercise, choose
activities that don't put
too much wear and tear
on your new hip.*

- Jogging and running

- High-impact exercise, such as aerobics

- Tennis

- Basketball

- Racquetball

- Contact sports, such as football

Follow-up visits

Your first follow-up visit to your doctor will be four to six weeks after you leave the hospital. (You may come back sooner to have your staples taken out.) At this time, the doctor will do a physical exam and make sure the wound is healing well. You may also have X-rays taken of your hip.

You will have more follow-up visits during the year to see how well you are doing. After the first year, most people can see their doctor once a year.

Preventing problems

After hip surgery, you need to watch for infections and other problems. Some of these problems could happen soon after surgery, while others might not show up until months or even years later.

Symptoms to watch for

Call your doctor right away if:

- Your leg is cool to the touch or a gray color.

- You feel numbness or tingling in your leg.

- You get a temperature of 101°F (38°C) or higher.

- You have chills.

- The area around the wound becomes more swollen, warm, red or painful.

- Fluid, pus or bright red blood comes out of the incision.

- You have increasing pain that is not helped by medicine, rest or ice packs.

- You notice a new or sudden swelling or pain in your thigh or calf.

- There is a burning feeling or foul odor when you urinate (go to the toilet), or you feel like you have to go more often than usual.

- You notice an unusual shortening or turning of your leg.

- You can't put weight on your leg (and you could before).

- You fall.

Preventing infection

If you get an infection caused by germs anywhere in your body, the germs could travel to your new hip. Though rare, an infection in your hip joint is a serious problem. The germs can settle around the new joint, and this may be hard to treat. Infection usually means you need more surgery.

Tip

From now on, you must take antibiotic medicine before having any dental work or medical procedure.

To prevent infection, you need to be extra careful from now on. If you get an illness, such as strep throat or pneumonia, tell your doctor right away. He or she will give you antibiotic medicine to stop the germs from spreading.

You will need to tell other care providers that you have had a joint replacement. This is true if you will have dental work or any type of surgery or procedure that may expose you to germs. You will need to take antibiotic medicine before having dental work or another procedure.

You will receive a medical alert card to carry in your wallet or billfold. In an emergency, this will tell care providers that you have an artificial hip.

Since an infection can develop in your hip joint many years after surgery, you will need to follow these rules all the time.

The key to recovery

Your doctors, nurses, therapists and other members of your care team want to do everything possible to give you a pain-free, working hip. But remember, you play a key role in the success of your hip replacement. You can increase the odds of a smooth recovery by having a positive attitude, doing your exercises every day, following your hip safety rules and watching for problems.

As the days go by, you will feel stronger, move more easily and have more energy. Then you can enjoy your new hip and the freedom it brings.

Having Your Hip Replaced . . . Again

Hip replacement surgery has an excellent track record—most people who have it will never need a second surgery. But sometimes, more surgery is the best option. Doctors may do a second surgery (called "revision surgery") if:

- Pain doesn't go away, even with pain pills and lifestyle changes.

- X-rays show damage to the new hip, such as bone loss, wearing of the surface or loosening of the joint.

- You break your hip.

- The ball pops out of the socket (dislocation).

- The joint becomes infected.

A second hip surgery is more difficult than the first one. The outcome is often not as good. For this reason, doctors explore other options before doing a second surgery.

Younger people who have a hip replaced are more likely to need a second surgery. That's because the new parts can wear out earlier, since younger people are often more active than older people.

Resources

American Academy of Orthopaedic Surgeons
6300 North River Road
Rosemount, Illinois 60018
Phone: 847-823-7186 or 800-824-AAOS [2267]
http://www.aaos.org
   The academy provides education and services for surgeons who treat disorders of the bones, joints, ligaments, muscles and tendons. It also provides information for patients.

American Association of Hip and Knee Surgeons
6300 North River Road, Suite 615
Rosemount, Illinois 60018
Phone: 847-698-1200
http://www.aahks.org/index.asp/fuseaction/patients.main
   The AAHKS provides information and education to surgeons as well as patients having hip or knee surgery. Provides information on minimally invasive surgery.

American Physical Therapy Association
1111 North Fairfax Street
Alexandria, Virginia 22314
Phone: 703-684-2782 or 800-999-2782
http://www.apta.org
   This national organization for physical therapists seeks to improve research, public understanding and education about physical therapy.

Arthritis Foundation
P.O. Box 7669
Atlanta, Georgia 30357
Phone: 404-872-7100
http://www.arthritis.org
   The foundation publishes pamphlets and other information for people who have arthritis.

Fairview Health Services
http://www.fairview.org

The Hip Society
c/o Karen Andersen
951 Old County Road, #182
Belmont, California 94002
Phone: 650-596-6190
http://www.hipsoc.org
   The society has a list of doctors who specialize in hip problems and provides information about hip problems.

National Institute of Arthritis and Musculoskeletal and Skin Diseases Information Clearinghouse
NIAMS/National Institutes of Health
1 AMS Circle
Bethesda, Maryland 20892
Phone: 301-495-4484 or 877-22-NIAMS [226-4267]
TTY: 301-565-2966
http://www.niams.nih.gov
   The clearinghouse provides information about various forms of arthritis and bone, muscle and skin diseases.

University of Minnesota Department of Orthopaedics
http://www.ortho.umn.edu
http://www.walkon.umn.edu

Glossary

abductor pillow: a triangle-shaped pillow that is placed between your legs to keep them from crossing

acetabulum: the round, cuplike part of the pelvis; the "socket" of the hip joint

acute pain: intense, severe pain that comes on suddenly

analgesic: pain medicine

anesthesia: medicine to remove sensation from all of the body (general anesthesia) or part of it (local anesthesia)

anti-inflammatory medications: drugs that reduce pain and swelling

arthritis: pain, swelling and stiffness in the joints

assistive device: walker, dressing stick, raised toilet seat or other item to help you do daily activities

cartilage: white or yellow tissue that connects parts of the body

catheter: a flexible tube that is put into the body to bring in or take out fluids

cement: a product used to attach the artificial joint to your bone. It works its way into the spaces in the bone, like cement between the bricks of a wall.

chronic pain: mild to severe pain that lasts a long time, usually more than two or three months

deep vein thrombosis (DVT): blood clots in the calf or thigh

dislocation: when the ball of the hip joint pops out of the socket, resulting in pain and limited movement

femur: thighbone

flexion limit: how much you can bend your hip

Hemovac: machine that collects the fluid from your wound after surgery

incentive spirometer: breathing machine that helps you to breathe deeply. It helps exercise your lungs and keep them clear.

incision: surgical cut or wound

infection: invasion of the body by harmful germs. Common symptoms of infection are pain, swelling and red, warm skin.

IV (intravenous) tube: a tube for putting fluids into a vein

loosening: when the artificial joint becomes detached or wears away from the bone

orthopedic surgeon: a surgeon who treats disorders of the bones and joints

osteoarthritis: "wear and tear" arthritis, marked by the wearing away of cartilage in the joint

OT: occupational therapy; provides help with daily activities such as dressing, using the toilet, bathing and household tasks

PCA pump: patient-controlled analgesia pump; a machine that gives pain medicine, which you control with a button

pelvis: bony structure at the lower part of the trunk; hipbones

PT: physical therapy; helps with exercises and your ability to move and walk

rehabilitation (rehab): physical therapy and occupational therapy

revision surgery: operation to replace the artificial hip

TEDs: white elastic socks used to prevent blood clots

weight-bearing status: how much weight you can put on your operated leg

Bibliography

Allina Health System. *Total Hip Replacement*. First edition. Minneapolis: Allina Press, 2004.

American Academy of Orthopaedic Surgeons. Minimally Invasive Hip Replacement. October 2004. At: http://www.orthoinfo.aaos.org/fact/thr_report.cfm?Thread_ID=471&topcategory=Hip.

———. Total Hip Replacement Exercise Guide. 2000. At: http://www.orthoinfo.aaos.org/booklet/view_report.cfm?Thread_ID=20&topcategory=Hip.

Fairview Health Services. *Before Your Surgery*. Minneapolis: Fairview Press, 2004.

———. "Minimally Invasive Hip Replacements: New Procedure Improves Recovery Period, Pain Management." *Inside Fairview-University Medical Center.* September 6, 2004.

———. *You and Your Total Hip Replacement*. Minneapolis: Fairview Health Services, 1997.

Grelsamer, Ronald P. *What Your Doctor May Not Tell You about Hip and Knee Replacement Surgery: Everything You Need to Know to Make the Right Decisions.* New York: Warner Books, 2004.

HealthLink (Medical College of Wisconsin). "With Minimally Invasive Hip Replacement, Less Is More." January 28, 2004. At: http://www.healthlink.mcw.edu/article/1031002336.html. Accessed October 20, 2004.

Healthpages.org. "A Patient's Guide to Total Hip Replacement Surgery." May 17, 1997. At: http://www.healthpages.org/ahp/library/hlthtop/thr/index.htm.

Mayo Clinic. "Advance Directives: Make Your Medical Care Wishes Known." July 16, 2003. At: http://www.mayoclinic.com/invoke.cfm?id=HA00014. Accessed January 25, 2005.

Mayo Clinic. "Total Hip Replacement: Relieve Pain, Improve Mobility." April 18, 2003. At: http://www.mayoclinic.com/invoke.cfm?id=9BE7ADB-2D2C-478908D784568379C6B70.

MedicineNet.com. "What Is a Total Hip Replacement?" February 2, 2003. At: http://www.medicinenet.com/script/main/art.asp?articlekey=497&pf=3&track=qup497.

Medline Plus Medical Encyclopedia. "Hip Joint Replacement." April 28, 2004. At: http://www.nlm.nih.gov/medlineplus/ency/article/002975. htm. Accessed May 20, 2005.

National Institute of Arthritis and Musculoskeletal and Skin Diseases. "Questions and Answers about Hip Replacement." NIH Publication No. 01-4907, n.d. At: http://www.niams.nih.gov/hi/topics/hip/ hiprepqa.htm. Accessed October 20, 2004.

Trahair, Richard. *All about Hip Replacement: A Patient's Guide.* Melbourne: Oxford University Press, 2000.

University of Virginia Health System. "Total Hip Replacement." November 19, 2002. At: http://www.healthsystem.virginia.edu:80/internet/ orthopaedics/thr.cfm. Accessed July 20, 2004.

University of Washington Department of Orthopaedics and Sports Medicine. "Surgical Options: 'Traditional' or 'Minimally-Invasive Hip Replacement?'" December 29, 2003. At: http://www.orthop. washington.edu/faculty/Leopold/hipreplacement/04. Accessed October 20, 2004.

———. "What Is Hip Replacement? A Review of Total Hip Arthroplasty, Hip Resurfacing, and Minimally-Invasive Hip Surgery," n.d. At: http:// www.orthop.washington.edu/faculty/Leopold/hipreplacement/print. Accessed October 20, 2004.

Virtual Hospital, University of Iowa Department of Orthopaedics. "Total Hip Replacement: A Guide for Patients." December 1999. At: http:// www.vh.org/adult/patient/orthopaedics/hipreplace/#2. Accessed July 20, 2004.